GU00976238

How to Analyze People with Dark Psychology

The Secrets to Speed Read People Like a Book, Defend Yourself and Influence Anyone Using Body Language, Persuasion, NLP, and Mind Control Techniques

(Emotional Intelligence Mastery, Book 1).

By

Charles P. Carlton

Disclaimer

This publication is designed to provide reliable information on the subject matter only for educational purposes, and it is not intended to provide medical advice for any medical treatment. You should always consult your doctor or physician for guidance before you stop, start, or alter any prescription medications or attempt to implement the methods discussed. This book is published independently by the author and has no affiliation with any brands or products mentioned within it. The author hereby disclaims any responsibility or liability whatsoever that is incurred from the use or application of the contents of this publication by the purchaser or reader. The purchaser or reader is hereby responsible for his or her own actions.

Books By The Same Author

How to Stop Overthinking (Change Your Life Series, Book 1)

Cognitive Behavioral Therapy Made Simple (Change Your Life Series, Book 2)

Master Your Emotions (2 Books in 1)

Stop Overthinking and Vagus Nerve Stimulation –

(2 Books in 1)

About The Author

Charles P. Carlton, a former consultant with a top big 4 global consulting firm, Ernst & Young and a Fortune 100 best companies to work for is a self-help professional, devoted to showing you the tricks on how to hack your life to get the most out of it by getting things done.

His quest for self-discovery led him to retire from the corporate world to fulfil his life-long goals of being a self-help coach and writer.

He specializes in using a cut-through science-based and personal experience approach in connecting with his audience in areas of emotional intelligence, self-esteem, and self-confidence, self-discovery, communication, personal development, and productivity. This has helped him build successful relationships and connections with his audience.

When not writing, Charles loves reading and exploring

the beauty of nature from where most times he gets many thought-provoking inspirations.

Table of Contents

Introduction

Have you ever been in this situation before?

You are seated before a person who you have been scheduled to meet with. It could be a business executive, a potential investor, or even a supposed friend whom you haven't seen in a while and who has requested to have a meeting with you.

You exchange pleasantries with this person who is seated at the other side of the table. You take a long look at him and one of the first things you can notice is that he reeks of affluence and influence. You can bet that the wide, glass table separating both of you is costlier than someone's annual salary. His firm grip on your hands as the both of you reach over the table for a handshake tells a story; this man is not one to be taken for granted and over the years, he has proven it with the empire he has built. His cologne fills the air and all you can tell from the scents that strike your senses is that the cologne is nothing but designers; possibly those limited-edition vials that are made for only the 1% of the world's most influential 10%.

You are supposed to be meeting with this man for a specific reason, and although he is smiling in your direction, you cannot shake the feeling that there is something off about the whole situation.

The chills that are crawling up your spine are too intense to be ignored, and before you can tell what is going on, you feel the trail of sweat as it rolls down from your armpits.

Is it the coldness of his deep voice?

Is it in the way his brown eyes seem to bore a hole into your skin, making you feel bare and exposed before him? Is it in the way that the smile on his mouth does not seem to be entirely genuine and does not light up his eyes?

You can't tell what it is. The only thing you are sure of is the fact that there is more to this man seated at the other side of the table; more to him than meets the eyes.

In no time, you hightail out of his office, thoughts of the weird encounter haunting you for the rest of the day.

Have you ever come in contact with people that were hard to read? These are the kinds of people that, although they may look polished and suave, you cannot shake that feeling that there may be some things you may be missing out on. They seem to set off all the warning bells in your head and make you feel spooked.

Every day presents itself with the opportunity to meet new people. Notwithstanding how you look at it and how much you may be trying to avoid it, you must make connections with people on an almost daily basis.

Whether you meet them virtually or physically, it does not change the fact that if you are going to be a highly successful person, you must be able to train yourself to be in tune with, and able to read people like a book. The ability to read cues that people give off subliminally, understand non-verbal communication, detect when someone is trying to keep something from you and protect yourself from people who may not have the best of interests for you is one of the key skills you must develop as a person who is on his way to becoming more successful.

It is with the knowledge of how important it is to protect yourself and be able to see past the facades that people present, that this book has been written on.

Within the next few chapters contained in this book, you will;

- Understand the concept of dark psychology and how you come in contact with it every day.
- Become aware of how those who are trained to make use of dark psychology wield these powers to ensure that they get what they want and when they want them.
- Understand how to analyze people and understand what their every body language means.
- You will find out the cues to look out for when interacting with people on a daily basis, what these cues could mean to you and how to improve your skills of non-verbal communication.

- Get to understand the concept and elements of persuasion, how it goes beyond just talking to people with your mouth alone and how you can discover when someone is trying to manipulate you into doing something.
- Gain some insights into Neuro-Linguistic Programming, what it means and how it relates to your everyday life.

- Discover tactics you can apply right away to defend yourself from manipulators.

And a whole lot more!

Whether you consider yourself to be a leader or not, a career person, a business owner, or just the regular Joe walking the streets every day, there is something for you within the following pages of this book. So, be sure you do not drop this book, but that you read it until you get to the last word and begin to work on all that you have learned. That is the only way through which you can unleash the power you will gain from getting exposed to the knowledge shared in this book.

Are you ready? Let's dive in.

Chapter 1

What is Dark Psychology?

To be able to understand the conversations we are about to have and better help you put things in the right perspective, let us begin this chapter with a story.

Some years back, there was a man who wanted to run for the office of the Presidency. He was so desperate that he began envisioning himself in the white house, seated on the chair of the president, with access to the president's quarters, his seal and his authority.

At the time he started having these dreams, there was a little problem.

He was working in the marketing and sales department of a design company and although it seemed as though he was doing well for himself, that was nothing compared to his ultimate dream of becoming the President (or at least getting himself into the White House and being in the close league of the President). Knowing this, he laid all the cards he had on the table and began taking inventory of all the skills in his arsenal.

By the time he was done with this step, he had discovered that he was a great public speaker and that over the years, he had been able to influence a good number of people just by talking to them in a group. As he was carrying out this exercise, he was able to recall many times that he had been sent by his bosses to speak to potential clients and investors because they had the utmost faith in him that all it took was for him to speak to them and they would be sold. Much to his delight, it dawned on him that all those times, their predictions had worked and all those clients had ended up doing business with them or investing in their firm.

He also discovered that in his toolbox of useful skills, he had the skill of being charismatic. As a choleric, he was considered to be the life of the party and a natural leader. Coupled with his speaking skills, he was able to make use of his ability to appear confident and on top of his game at all times to convince people into doing what he wanted them to, charm them into thinking that his thoughts were the best and if not done his way, things would go out of control. While on this soul-searching spree, he discovered a lot about himself, and as such, the journey to the White House began.

It took a lot of years, but he was able to start forming the right connections that he needed. It required that he moved over to a bigger city, and given the odds of what he wanted happening for him there, he knew he had no option than to answer the call of his destiny. After a few long years of working day and night, he was able to make it to the floor of the senate, where he delivered a rousing speech before the members of the senate. In no time, he was appointed to become a Senator of state, and that was just the beginning of the life he wanted to live and create for himself.

Whether or not he ended up as the President, sitting in the White House and with all that power under his belt is something you would have to figure out for yourself. But from the little you have deduced about this goal-driven, daredevil man, what do you think it will be?

Why did we have to tell this story, you may ask.

The truth is this; this man was able to achieve his dream (or the part that you saw him achieve) because of a lot of things. Asides the fact that he strongly believed it was his destiny to become a highly placed person in society, he was able to pick up and deploy skills that were instrumental toward making sure that he got to where he wanted to be. One of these was his ability to communicate with people in such a way that struck a chord so deep in their heart, influence them to do things they would not have ordinarily done and get them to buy into his ideologies.

This is the entirety of the concept of dark psychology.

So, in essence, dark psychology is the art and science of manipulation and mind control. When put that way, it seems all magical and completely evil and while there are dark sides to this, it is not all doom and gloom either. Let's throw a little light on this, shall we?

Dark Psychology is the phenomenon by which people use various tactics, including motivation, persuasion, manipulation and coercion in order to get what they want. What this implies is that dark psychology begins from the point of clearly understanding what a person wants and the things he must do in order to get him what he wants. Then he must go ahead to make use of all the elements listed above in places they are necessary to get him to achieve the things he has set out for himself. If you take a close look at the elements listed above, you will see that dark psychology is something you encounter on a daily basis, from the person trying to sell his brand to you and get you to patronize his business, to the one who tries to motivate you to get you up and going with your life. You really cannot turn away from dark psychology.

Before we get ahead of ourselves, let us touch on a few basis of dark psychology, shall we?

Evolutionary Psychology: The Human Dark Side

Over the years, it has been proven that the heart of man is not all shades of amazing. Religious books like the Bible and the Qur'an clearly point out in various places that human beings are prone to acting badly at times. This may not be that they want to be bad, but it could stem from the fact that there is a predisposition towards being bad that has been placed in the nature of man. This is exactly how the Qur'an puts it;

"I do not exculpate myself. Lo! The (human) soul enjoineth unto evil, save that, whereon my Lord hath mercy." (Surah Yusuf 12:53).

In more modern renditions of this verse of the Qur'an, and in places it has been drawn upon in order to buttress different points in modern context, the word *enjoineth* has been replaced with the phrase *to be prone to*. This implies that man has that tendency to drift off the path he knows he should be walking – the path of good and what is right – to walk the path of wrong, driven by his desires and the things that he may want to get.

The Bible also confirms that this is the case with man. In the exact words that were used in the Bible, *"the heart of man is deceitful above all things, and desperately wicked: who can know it?"* (Jeremiah 17:9). Many times, the Bible throws light on the fact that there is a part of man that is given to mischief and that there is the tendency for man to go the wrong way and do things he is not supposed to do.

This is the knowledge of the Dark Side of Human Nature.

Over the years, it became glaring that if left unattended, this dark side tended to overshadow the good in man and the result of this is that man is going to be turned into a beast. The need for this dark side to be illuminated and taken away from man increased over the years, giving psychologists and other scientists a reason to begin a series of studies to help them achieve what they wanted to achieve.

As studies went on, the concept of Evolutionary Psychology was introduced. In a nutshell, evolutionary Psychology is the part of psychology that has been used to illuminate the dark and shadowy sides of human nature. Evolutionary Psychology can help shed light on a range of human behavior and it is quite helpful as you journey towards answering the question, *"why do you do what you do?"* Just like almost every other scientific process, evolutionary psychology draws on the assumptions that your mind, just like every other part of your body, has adapted and evolved over time. It tries to contrast the degree of this evolution to the way you live your life and how you respond to the things that happen around you.

In a nutshell, evolutionary psychology is considered to have the answer to the question of why you act the way you do because it studies a host of parameters and begins to draw conclusions with regards to your behavior; finding the parallels between the dark sides of your nature and trying to shed light on them.

Tactics Used in Dark Psychology

As hinted in the sections above, dark psychology can be considered to be a school that offers a range of courses. This implies that there are a lot of components and tactics that make up what we know as dark psychology, and these components come into play as people make use of them to get what they want on a daily basis.

Here are a few of these tactics.

1. **Manipulation;** While this may seem as though it is too hideous to be spoken of, every one of us has a part of us that has made use of this tactic before to get what we wanted. This is what happens when a child decided to throw tantrums in order to get his parent to buy him a toy that he wants, or even when a person decides that the easiest way for him to get the cooperation of another person to achieve a goal is by blackmailing the person. You have made use of some elements of manipulation before, but the difference usually lies in the degree to which you manipulate people, and to what end you are trying to manipulate them.

   Having this in mind, it is necessary that we understand what manipulation is all about. Manipulation is the practice of manipulating or the state of being manipulated. To manipulate means to influence, manage, direct, control, or to tamper with something. When you take a closer look at the words that have been used to explain the concept of manipulation, you will see that, to some extent, you must have made use of a few of these elements to get you to your desired end at some point in time. However, the goal of this book is to make sure that you are enriched with the right knowledge that will help you detect when someone is trying to pull this stunt on you and help you with practical ways to counter the effect of his efforts.

Manipulation, in most cases, does not present itself as manipulation. You will hardly ever see someone walk up to you and tell you that he is on a mission to manipulate you or get you to do something that you are not willing to do. It is usually a gradual process and demands a lot of precision in order for it to work. As a result of this fact, there are a lot of ways in which manipulation can present itself in your everyday life.

2. **Charm;** Have you ever met someone who is so fluid and oozes a lot of charm? He is the person who knows all the right words to say at all the

right times and does not hesitate to say all of them. He is the one who can press all the right buttons and he makes sure he achieves this. According to the dictionary, charm is the ability to persuade, delight or arouse admiration.

This tactic speaks to the sensual part of a person. People who make use of this tactic believe that once they find someone who they need a favor from, all they need to do is try to act a bit flirty. The result of the new trajectory of their actions is that the object of their attention begins to become a bit relaxed around them and in due time, they end up getting what they want. This tactic is seen more in the corporate world, especially when someone is trying to get into a position he is not yet meant and equipped for.

3. **Coercion;** The first thing you must note about coercion is that it is not always fun. This involves some amount of brute force and in most cases, it is not sweet to be coerced into doing something. Coercion is the act of making use of threatened

force in order to compel another person to take a decision to carry out an action that he would not have otherwise carried out. It goes without saying that, in most cases, coercion goes against the use of free will because those that are coerced do not always have the luxury of making choices.

Coercion banks on fear; the fear of harm or threats. In this tactic, the person who is perpetrating the act paints the picture that it is better to carry out the action he wants the person he is forcing to carry out because the consequences of not being a part of what he wants him to get involved in can be very severe. For example, if someone is being coerced into being an accomplice for a crime, the person doing the coercion will make the coerced know that he will be killed if he does not agree to be a part of what is going on. Since the other person who is being coerced sees his life as being more important to lose, he would rather decide to get involved and not think of the consequences.

4. **The silent treatment;** Inasmuch as this seems as though it should not be here, you will be shocked to discover that it is a manipulation tool that is as effective as any other tool that we will be discussing in this section of the book. Mostly, the silent treatment works on those that have a close relationship with others and have, over the years, built a stream of communication and trust between themselves.

The person giving the cold shoulder through silent treatment banks on the assumption that the other person can almost not do without reaching out to him. So, when the silent treatment starts, the other party has no option than to listen to what he is saying because he won't be able to bear the disconnection in communication between the both of them. This silent treatment builds up the anxiety between them, and in no time, the person on the receiving end of the silent treatment may be forced to call a truce.

5. **Appeal to reason;** Although we cannot say that all manipulation and dark psychology tactics are negative, what we know is that even those that are not bad in themselves can be used in a wrong way. In this type of tactic, the person who is looking to get his way makes use of a logical argument or tries to appeal to the sense of the logic of the other person. He makes an argument that is not wrong in itself, but when looked at from the lens of context, it won't be ethically right either.

For example, if a student decides to break into the office of a school authority in order to obtain the questions for their examinations, he can try getting someone to be his accomplice and to do this, he can make use of the argument – " remember, if you help me get this, you will be graduating with your mates this year given how poorly you have performed in quizzes and assignments." While the argument is not wrong in itself, when looked at from the lens of context, it is not ethical to break into an office to gain firsthand knowledge of examination questions. However, the logic behind the offer will most likely drive the other person into agreeing to do what he wants him to do.

6. **Self-abasement;** This tactic works on the person who is using it. It goes without saying that not all dark psychology tactics work on the other person; this is an example of such tactics that the user directs towards himself while expecting a reaction from the other person.

This is how self-abasement works.

Imagine that someone is looking to obtain something from you, maybe seeking forgiveness or trying to make a relationship stronger after doing something wrong. Still angry and you have decided you are not about to forgive him anytime soon. Then one day, he walks up to you and after trying to apologize for the umpteenth time, launches into a tirade where he seems to turn against himself with hurtful words like "it is all my fault," "I always ruin everything," "just my dumb luck."

If this person is able to pull this off well, you most likely will begin to let your guard down. Instead of sticking to the plan you have made before this time, you will see that your defenses will begin to crack and in no time, you will give in to whatever the person wanted you to do. Self-abasement usually works in hand with regression, which is also a tactic that people use when they want to get their way. Regression is basically when an adult starts behaving like a child in order to get what he wants out of another person. For example, when an adult begins to wail or throw tantrums, it usually becomes too embarrassing that the other person has no choice but to give in to what he wants to be done.

7. **Hardball;** This is a form of manipulation. Although other forms of manipulation would usually threaten that something will happen if the other party does not have his way, anyone

making use of this tactic will actually cause you bodily harm in order to get what he wants. So, if he requests that you do something and you refuse, he will make sure that he does something to you that will harm you. This way, you get scared of what he could possibly do next and give in to what he wants. This is the skill that bullies use to get those they are bullying to keep up with whatever they want from them.

8. **Motivation;** As we have said earlier, not all forms of dark psychology are bad in themselves. It all depends on the context of use. While motivation is a great tool that is employed by leaders to achieve great feats, it is also a weapon of mass destruction if used by the wrong person and under the wrong circumstances.

Motivation is the art of employing different strategies, including speaking to people in order to get them charged up to do something they may not have ordinarily done. For example, if a lecturer tells his students that to be successful and to amount to anything good, hard work and diligence must be their daily anthem, and he does this in such a way that the students connect with what he is saying and feel energized to take their academics more seriously, he has not only advised them but has motivated them to do something they would have found difficult if left on their own. On the other hand, another person can make use of this skill in the wrong way.

For example, a leader who encourages his followers to give themselves and their safety up to fight a battle he knows they are ultimately going to lose. With his skill of motivation, he may decide to speak to the people and make them see many reasons why they need to fight. While it is not bad for them to take a stand, he will take advantage of his influence over them and make them get the result he wants them to get. This is one of the skills that leaders in the war front use to get their men into a fighting spirit. They do this because they don't want to get into a fight and lose their lives out of fear.

Dark Psychology Tricks

Asides the tactics and forms of dark psychology we discussed in the section above, there are a few tricks that people have pulled off in times past just to get their way. If you are observant enough, you will find a number of them that have been used on you. As said earlier, part of the aim this book seeks to accomplish is to equip you with the knowledge to guard yourself with when people try to pull these stunts on you.

Here are a few of these tricks;

1. **Hardly evil;** Zig Ziglar made a quote that has been handed down over the years. He says, "if you can help advance someone's goals, then you can get all you want in life." This is one of the tricks that those who make use of dark psychology use in order to get what they want.

    This trick banks on the knowledge that humans tend to be selfish; they put themselves and personal interests above and before everything else. With this knowledge, a person can help you achieve your goals not because he likes you per se, but because he is doing it with hopes that you will soon see the need to do him a favor in return. This trick is addressed as hardly evil because of the fact that it appears to be seemingly harmless, and everyone tends to pull it off at some point in their lives. This trick is used in the business and corporate world, and even in people's personal lives. For example, if someone is moving to be promoted to the position of the CEO of an organization, it is only normal to see that there would usually be those people around him who will be very instrumental toward getting him what he wants, with the hopes that once he assumes that position officially, they won't be left behind in any way.

2. **Blatant manipulation;** This trick is used when someone is trying to get you to like them almost immediately. In this trick, the person subtly begins to mirror you in everything they do. So, if both of you are having a conversation, you will discover that the person will begin to mimic you, genuflect the way you are, mirror your poise and

even begin to make their voice sound a bit like yours. The result of this is that you may begin to feel a bit at ease, and in no time, he would have worked his way into your heart.

The challenge with this trick is that it is a double-edged sword. While it may work on some people, it may not work on others because they may see this trick as trying to send them signals that they are not good enough and the result of this perception is that the person closes off and becomes shifty.

3. Another trick that is used in dark psychology is the trick of **holding off on making requests** until the person who should grant the request is tired, overwhelmed or completely distracted. This trick has been used by many to get what they want without a lot of stress or challenges. When a person is tired or feeling overwhelmed, the parts of his brain, which process information, seem to become slow to work. The result of this is that the person is more inclined to making spontaneous

decisions, and in most cases, will do anything just to make sure that nothing disturbs him or sets him off the more. It is at this point that the other person who wants to get something done swoops in and gets away with what he wanted.

For example, a child who waits until his father is tired before asking him to sign the permit for a field trip his father would not have signed if he were to be agile and attentive. There are many other instances and occasions where this trick is used by some persons to get what they want, especially if they know that they would not get it otherwise. This trick banks on the knowledge that when people are worn out, they are more likely to agree with anything that offers them some kind of respite, even if that thing is what they would not have ordinarily done.

4. **Terror induction;** People will do anything to escape terror and the impending fear of something bad happening to them. This trick is hinged on this knowledge, and many companies

and businesses make use of this knowledge to advertise their products/services in order to sell to the public.

The trick is simple. The person who wants to get something out of another person gets to achieve this by scaring the other person. When the person is afraid of what could possibly happen, he swoops in and gets what he really wants out of them. For example, a company that sells insurance plans for cars and houses can adopt this trick. All they need to do is paint a picture of what could happen if you are to lose your house and car to an accident. While you are yet reeling from the fear of losing your house and your car, and calculating the amount of money and time it will take you to build another one or purchase another car, they introduce their insurance plan. Because you are already scared of what would happen if you do not get on board, you will be more likely inclined towards getting the insurance plan. This is one very handy business trick.

5. **Confusion;** The rule of this trick is simple; "confuse people to get them to agree with you and accept whatever you tell them." When someone tries to apply this trick, you will discover that he may begin to;

- Speak at a rate that is too fast for you to follow through immediately.
- Speak of things that are disconnected and do not make any sense together.

You must understand that the intention of that person would usually be to confuse you with a lot of information, and when they sense that your brain is beginning to get overwhelmed with all that is being said to you, they slip in a request. At this point, there is every tendency that you will agree to whatever request they make, not because you want to, but because your mind was in a state where processing information was almost impossible for you.

As a way to make sure that you never fall into this trap, never try to make major decisions whenever you are feeling overwhelmed. Instead, it will do you a lot of good if you can wait and clear your head before you make those decisions. As much as it lies within you, allow the person to wait and promise him that you will send feedback when you are in a better emotional and psychological state.

Understanding the Dark Triad of Personality

As we established earlier, there is a dark side in every individual and this dark side constantly seeks to overshadow the good side of people. However, as psychology and the study of human behavior began to evolve, psychologists began to discover that there is more to this than what they thought.

The term was coined in early 2002, and it was adopted to speak of a set of three interconnected character traits that are a measure of how predisposed a person will be towards being bad. These three are a set of unusually connected and very negative traits that can cause lethal harm in all relationships, especially intimate relationships. These traits are; Narcissism, Psychopathy, and Machiavellianism. Individually, these traits are bad, but when combined, they produce an effect that is deadly, to say the least.

Narcissism

Narcissism is an exceptional love for oneself, especially when it is considered to be unhealthy and lethal towards others. Everyone is expected to love themselves, but when this love gets to a point where it is as though the person has a health issue, and just cannot get over the fact of how awesome and amazing he is, then it may be that he is battling with this illness.

This is characterized by the following;

- The pursuit of ego and its satisfaction. The narcissist can do anything to ensure that his ego remains untouched. His sense of self-respect can never take a beating and this is not in a good way of someone having a great sense of self-esteem. The narcissist sees every kind of challenge or confrontation (even the good-natured ones that should lead to growth and learning) as an opportunity staged by the other person to ridicule him, and he does not tend lightly to these things.

- The narcissist believes in perfection, although this has been proven over time to be nothing but an illusion. The narcissist believes that he is the spitting image of perfection, from his looks to his mannerisms and his work ethics. His mantra is that nothing can go wrong as far as he is the one that has done it, or as far as it concerns him. While self-confidence is a great tool that ensures you always remain at the top of your game, this is also not self-confidence because it is done to unhealthy levels. If another person sees a fault with whatever the narcissist does, he is more likely to throw a hissy fit in order to prove that the other party is wrong, or depending on how intense he perceives the matter to be, he can even pull a dagger and get into a fight.

- The narcissist feels entitled. Because of the emotions he has bottled up within and all the thoughts that pass through his mind on a daily basis, the narcissist feels entitled to whatever he wants. He does not understand the concept of making a request because he feels that he is doing the other person a favor by asking. When he needs something from you, you either provide it or be prepared for him to obtain it through whatever means he deems fit.

As you can see, narcissism shares some of the traits that are needed for your growth, and this is what makes it dangerous. It can be difficult to spot this trait, but when it is spotted, the person needs urgent professional help and intervention because he is like a ticking time bomb.

Psychopathy

This is a severe personality disorder that is characterized by a repeated pattern of lying, exploitation, the inability to listen to warnings and instruction, excessive arrogance, low or non-existent self-control, sexual indiscipline, and the inability to feel for others or be remorseful when the person commits a crime.

Considering that this is a personality disorder, the person who suffers from this is less likely to get a physical cure, but the best line of action is to take him to the professionals who handle psychological problems and let them work their magic on him.

A psychopath is very dangerous because of a number of reasons. Here are a few things that may be indicative of psychopathy;

- The psychopath is uncharacteristically callous and selfish. He derives so much joy whenever he gets his way and it does not matter if the other party is in severe pain or even dies as a result of his decisions. All he wants is all that happens – at every time.
- The psychopath is known for being spontaneous in his actions and decisions. He does not understand what it means to think things through, and he has the tendency to go off on the first wave of emotions that hit him as far as any matter is concerned. If the first wave is to draw

the daggers and leave a trail of dead bodies in his wake, so be it.

- The psychopath is usually an anti-social person. He does not have a lot of friends, and the result of this is that he has ample time to think up and conjure a million cunning schemes. His lack of friends and a lot of social entanglements can be as a result of the fact that he is quite unpredictable, and may have a history of having hissy fits and temper tantrums. Since not a lot of people will be willing to be in the face of that, the psychopath has to be on his own most of the time. This is a double-edged sword and hardly does any good in the long run.
- The psychopath is not left alone, either. It is not unusual to notice that the psychopath derives joy in making himself suffer pain. He believes that there is no gain until there is pain, and he takes this literally. He can be prone to inflicting bodily injuries on himself.

Psychopathy is not a trait that should be swept under the carpet. If, at any point, you notice that there is any person who is showing these signs, do well to get him help as soon as you can.

Machiavellianism

This is another severe case, more like a desperate measure in which a person makes use of extreme manipulation, ruthless behaviors and devious means to get what he wants. As we said in this book, everyone tends to pull a few stunts (a few, relatively harmless stunts) when they want something from someone who does not seem to be so eager to let them have it, but this is on the other side of the charts. A Machiavellian achieves his goals by cunning ways, crafting schemes that are too devious and can resort to the use of brute force when the going gets tough.

For example, the leader who decides that he is going to detain and make a practice of killing people just to obtain a piece of information from them is making use of this practice. The Machiavellian;

- Has an extremely warped sense of right and wrong. He does not see life as white or black, good or bad, yin or yang. All he sees are shades of grey, and many times he does not understand the concept of limits. The Machiavellian leader has little or no respect for the human rights of his followers as he would do anything to get what he wants.

- The Machiavellian is highly intelligent or does all he can to appear as a person of intelligence. If he is going to be able to pull off all the stunts he has planned to pull off, and influence people to move in the direction he wants them to move, he has to be a few steps ahead of the rest. This person understands the place of intelligence, and he does not hesitate to get his hands on any material or tool that will make him appear more intelligent or keep him abreast most of the time.

When these traits are considered in isolation, they are terrible. But if they are found to be present in the same person at the same time, the combination is ghastly, and this is what gives rise to the alarm with which the concept of psychological dark triad is addressed. People who score high on this scale have been proven to be more inclined towards crime, and they are the ones that usually create severe problems for an organization or society. If a person who has scored high on this scale, or has shown these signs over a sustainable period of time ascend to a position of authority in any sphere, he is more likely to create a lot of problems for the system, and if not checked, this can be a life-threatening situation.

Everyday Users of Dark Psychology

As we have pointed out time and again, you interact with dark psychology on a daily basis. Almost every person you interact with makes use of these skills to try and get something out of you. The degrees to which they make use of these skills differ, and the intents that are behind their actions are not all the same. However, this does not change the fact that you should be aware of what is happening at all times, so you can be able to spot out when a person is making use of dark psychology on you, and how to immune yourself from these tactics.

Politicians

Politicians are probably the greatest users of dark psychology. If you are to take an inventory of all the dark psychology skills and tactics, you will discover that the very successful politician has, at some point, made use of a good number of these skills to get his way with the people.

Starting from motivation to persuasion and all forms of subtle manipulation, the successful politician is more likely to make use of this skill to work his way into the hearts of the people. If he is looking to get people to love him, respect him and be on his side, he would have to learn how to get them to buy into his ideas and concepts. To achieve this, he needs the skill of motivation, and he even needs to persuade them to come aboard his dreams and visions. The politician must be able to get people to like him within the shortest possible time, and to achieve this, he will most likely make use of any of the tactics discussed in the sections above. There are a lot of reasons why the politician has to resort to making use of dark psychology, but it matters to what degree he makes use of these skills.

Salespeople

If the salesman is going to hit his marketing and sales goals, he will have to employ one or more of these tactics that have been discussed. Can you cast your mind back a bit and remember the last time a man selling his wares met you on the road and ended up convincing you to get something you had absolutely no need of? If you can, can we make an inventory of all the skills he used?

His powers of persuasion were intact, or else he would not have been able to get you to buy what you would not have ordinarily bought. Another skill he most likely made use of was the skill of motivation. There most likely was that time when you were not interested in getting what he was selling. Maybe you had decided after all that what he was selling was unnecessary or that you could do without it for the meantime. At this point, he most likely dug into his bag of skills and pulled out motivation. In no time, you ended up getting that product he was trying to sell to you. A company can likewise include terror in their marketing strategy. As we discussed earlier, they can get you to be scared with their adverts. Under these conditions, their ads are geared toward making sure that you see what you will be missing out on if you do not jump on the bandwagon and purchase their product or service.

All these are forms of dark psychology, used to make different ends meet.

Religious or Cult leaders

Let us establish this fact immediately; all leaders make use of these skills at some point or the other. Religious leaders and heads of cult groups and sects are not exempted from the use of these skills. Most public speakers (those that have to speak to many people at the same time and influence their thoughts and actions) buy into these skills to get their message across. Religious leaders and the heads of cult groups fall into the category of public speakers, and they have to rely on most of these skills to be able to get the messages they have across to their audience, get the people to buy into their concepts and also get them to trust them. To achieve his, they use motivation, persuasion, and in some cases, terror to achieve their aims.

Sociopaths

Sociopaths are people who are antisocial in their behavior. They exhibit antisocial behaviors, which include the fear of social interaction, an aversion to public gatherings, and so on. These people prefer to be holed up in their own end of the world, rather than go out and make friends or be with people that they have established a deep connection with overtime. Under extreme situations, sociopaths completely disregard other people, and this results in an unhealthy relationship with people.

In order to get their way whenever they want to, they make use of a number of skills. These are the ways through which sociopaths achieve their aims;

- They resort to making use of blatant force to get their way with whoever they want to. As discussed above, they have little or no regard for other people and as such, they are not interested in the health and safety of others. It wouldn't mean much to them if they are to draw the sword and resort to causing others bodily harm.

- They make use of manipulation to have their way. This can come in the form of pleasure induction, the threats of pain, and every other manipulative process that they can pull off.

- They adopt the use of too many words and ambiguous phrases. The goal of this is to get you to start feeling overwhelmed while they mask vital information about what they are doing from you. This is a practical example of where confusion comes into play, and it is your duty to spot it out and nip it in the bud.

Attorneys

Attorneys and lawyers, in general, make use of these skills to achieve their ends. Because they have to make convincing arguments in court, dig deeper than the surface to see the things that the regular person may not see and take decisions that may be too difficult for the normal person, they have to make use of some of these skills to get to their ends. The lawyer has to;

- Persuade people to give them information that they ordinarily wouldn't have divulged. To achieve this, they must be able to convince them to work with him.
- They can also make use of terror induction when the time calls for it. Under some circumstances, they may not be as willing to divulge secrets as they should be, but to get them to cooperate, the lawyer can make use of this skill.

Selfish people

Selfish people make use of all these skills to have their way. It is usually an interplay of all the dark psychology secrets they can lay their hands on, and they hardly ever pay attention to the effects their activities have on other people. If you are to take an inventory of all the tricks we have discussed, you may discover that these people make use of all of them.

The selfish person who decides that he is going to rob a bank can decide to get you onboard his plan by making use of one or more of these strategies;

- The silent treatment, especially if you are close and shared a relationship where there was a lot of communication.
- Manipulation, by employing any of the strategies discussed above.
- Terror induction, and the fear that comes with the knowledge that the person can cause you bodily harm at any point.

This category of people should be looked out for because they hardly ever consider the effects of what they are doing as it has to do with others. Coupled with narcissists, selfish people rank the highest in the classes of those that are more likely to make use of dark psychology to get what they want.

How Manipulative People Uses Dark Psychology to Control Others

As we have hinted in the sections above, dark psychology is something that many people in today's world make use of in order to get what they want at all times. Although it is not always easy to spot out manipulation, if you are trained to spot the characteristics, you will see them in time and be able to block them out. Here are a few practical ways that manipulative people try to achieve their aims, a few we have already touched on;

- Self-abasement. The person manipulating can resort to making use of words and expressions that make him appear to be less valuable than he truly is. The aim of these is to make sure that you see that he is helpless, and try to appeal to your sense of pity/compassion. Look out for these in your everyday interactions with people and learn how to stick to the decisions you have made, even if the other person is trying to pull this stunt on you.

- A skilled manipulator is perfect in the art of making "turning tables" in their favor. They make sure that they are perceived as the ones who ate at the receiving end of the hurt and pain, regardless of whether or not this is the truth. A manipulating partner always resorts to making it appear as though the other partner is the one at fault, and he is very vocal at doing this. In this scenario, you will hear statements like, "you are causing me a lot of harm," "can't you see I am hurting?" and all the rest of them. This person hardly ever pays attention to the other partner, because it is all about him.

- The manipulative person waits for you and only strikes when he knows that you are not at your best. This could be when you are at your weakest, unhappy or generally not in the mood to be pressurized about anything. These are the times this person will make requests of you. Because you are not in the place to think as critically as you are supposed to, or make informed decisions, there is every tendency that he will get his way with you.

- Manipulative people play on your fears. They latch on to that thing that they know you are highly afraid of, and with this thing, they can get you to do their bidding for a very long time. For example, a person who wants to manipulate another into doing what is unethical will most likely threaten or manipulate that person into doing this by making use of the person's worst fears; maybe the fear of losing a loved one or exposing something he would rather keep a secret.

Traits of Manipulative People

Here are a few red flags that you should look out for when relating to people. These are indicators that a person is manipulative;

1. Manipulators play the role of being the victim very well. They achieve this because they are skilled at portraying themselves as innocent.

2. These people are professionals in playing the guilt card. They cash in on others' empathy and sense of indebtedness to them and they exploit these. If you fail to give in to every one of the manipulator's demands, he will find a way to make sure that you never get over the guilt for a very long time. During that period of time when you are battling guilt, you will end up doing so much more for them than you can possibly think of.

3. They are overly self-centered. All their thoughts and actions revolve around themselves, and they do all they can to make sure that the people in their spheres of influence see them as the most important figures in their lives.

4. Manipulative people are bullies. They would not hesitate to resort to bullying if they perceive it to be the only way through which they can get you to do what they want you to.

5. They make use of a lot of verbal jabs, innuendos and covert insults to get their way. The

manipulative person knows just what to say, when to say it and under what conditions it must be said to get you to react in a certain way. These people are skilled in the art of using words, and they wield this tool with a lot of precision. Manipulative people are abusive. They do not mind making use of all the tools they have at their disposal to get what they want, even if these tools are borderline abusive and very lethal to the other person or people involved.

Key Points from Chapter One

- Dark psychology is the use of various tactics, including motivation, persuasion, manipulation and coercion in order for people to get what they want.

- At some point or the other, you have made use of these skills to achieve an aim for yourself. It does not make you a bad person. However, the difference between the people who use this in a bad way and those who use it in ways that are not lethal to others per se, is the knowledge of healthy boundaries and a commitment to remain within these boundaries.

- The dark triad of psychology includes; Narcissism, Psychopathy and Machiavellianism. These are a measure of how much a person is inclined towards being bad, and a person who shows these symptoms or checks all these boxes should be taken for immediate professional attention.

- You will see users of dark psychology as you interact with people on a daily basis. Your primary assignment is to arm yourself with the skills and the knowledge you will get from this book in order to make sure that they do not get the best of you.

Chapter 2

Analyzing People through Body Language

The Psychology of Body Language

Let's play a little game of guessing, shall we?

You most likely have been in a conversation or deep interaction with someone before now and during the course of the conversation, something you could not quite place your hands on felt off.

Although the person may have been responding to what you were saying, you could not help but pick up those signs that there was something that was not quite right about the conversation. He may have been nodding and may have even had that too-broad-to-be-believed smile stretching out on his face, but you could not place your hands on what was wrong.

So, you had no option than to do what you felt was best to be done at the moment; you ended the conversation so the both of you could go your separate ways.

In retrospect, can you point out what it was that made the flow of that conversation seem forced to you? Can you tell what it was that yelled to your senses that the person had better things to do than listen to you? You may not be able to answer these questions immediately, and that is what makes what we are about to discuss more important to the success of your relationships with people.

Before we proceed, let us take a look at what body language is all about.

Wikipedia defines body language as a type of non-verbal communication in which physical behaviors (as opposed to words) are used to express or convey information. Body language includes a lot of elements ranging from facial expressions, body postures, gestures and touch, to the use of physical spaces. In this section of the book, we will take a look at this tool and why it is almost as effective (if not more effective than) the use of words in conveying a person's true feelings and emotional state at every time.

In order to be able to fully understand people and the messages they try to pass across to you per second, you must have an eye that is attentive to details and can be able to understand body language. According to psychologists and the specialists that study social interactions and how man interacts with others in today's social context, body language is a silent orchestra as people constantly give clues as to what they are thinking of and feeling at every point. [Body Language (Psychology Today International)].

The psychology of body language comes into play when body language is picked up and processed by others in order to ascertain what the person who gives off those signals may be truly feeling per time. As science has proven, most body language signals are given off unconsciously, and as a result of this, they are considered to be a more accurate mirror of what a person is thinking or feels about a situation. When you are able to understand this, you will be able to 'read' people, and this is one skill that is required as you journey to becoming more precise in how you relate with people.

Inasmuch as body language can play a pivotal role in helping you have an insight into how people feel at every point, it is not always a very accurate index to measure whether or not someone is receptive to what he is receiving at every given time. This is because the more people get exposed to the way things work in the world, the more they understand how body language can be interpreted and as a result, they can train themselves to control their body language, thereby making others see and believe what is not entirely correct. This implies that body language can be controlled by sheer force and willpower.

Why Non-Verbal Communication Matters

1. Non-verbal communication can be a very handy tool to help you increase the amount of trust and faith people have in you. When people discover that your non-verbal communication and what you are saying with your mouth tally, they become more inclined to trust and accept you with all their hearts. This is because they will begin to perceive you as being honest and not trying to hide anything away from them.

2. Non-verbal communication is a very viable way of passing across information without having to make use of one's vocal cords. For example, in a condition when it is not a good idea for one to speak (maybe under duress or other bad scenarios), such a person can rely on these non-verbal cues to pass his messages across to the people that must receive them. He can choose from any of the methods of non-verbal communication that are available to him.

3. Non-verbal communication is an ingrained part of social interactions. As we discussed earlier, everybody gives off these cues knowingly and unknowingly. Knowing this, you will be able to understand that although non-verbal communication is a great tool that can help you gain the trust of people much faster, it can also be a tool that will make people lose their ability to trust you. If a person sees you as someone who is not as genuine as he poses to be (this happens when what you are saying is different from the cues they are picking up from your non-verbal

communication), they would most likely be tempted to pass you off as someone who is not to be trusted. This can take a bad toll on your relationships and the success of your career in the long run.

Types of Non-Verbal Communication

There are several types of non-verbal communication. The most commonly used of them all include;

1. **Facial expressions;** As the name implies, this is a collective name given to all the expressions that flit across your face under a given circumstance. Considering the anatomy of the human face (which includes the facial muscles and the facial nerve), the human face is a highly expressive part of the human anatomy. The result of this expressiveness is that the face is able to convey a lot of information that the mouth fails to convey.

   For example, a downward turn of the corners of the lips will usually imply that the person who has this expression on his face may be annoyed, irritated or simply bored by whatever is going on, whether or not he may accept it. Also, when a person smiles, this expressive nature of the face makes it possible for another to be able to tell whether the smile is genuine or not. A genuine smile touches the side of the eyes, causing the muscles that surround the eyes to crinkle, and a glint to come up from the eyes. This is one of the easiest ways to know if a person is really pleased, and this is only possible because of the expressive nature of the face.

2. **Touch and the concept of physical space;** Something as minute and overlookable as a touch can carry a lot of messages within it. This is why you need to understand the signals that people get from touch and know how to make use of this knowledge to pass across pieces of information that match with what you really want to pass across.

Take the following examples into consideration;

A slight pat on the shoulders can mean acceptance or concession, a weak handshake can be used to send signals that the person giving the handshake may not be up for some kind of confrontation, and a bear hug can mean that the person who is giving it means a lot of goodwill for the person he is giving the hug to. Even those who want to make passes at others in a sexual way usually resort to making use of this type of non-verbal communication to pass their messages across. They most likely start using cues like taking every opportunity to touch the other person and getting in his personal space as a sign that they are interested in him romantically or otherwise.

3. **Gestures and posture;** Your posture and the way you make use of your hands when you speak or interact with people can carry a lot of interpretation and meaning for the other party. For example, when a person folds his arms over his chest, it could imply that he may be mentally preparing himself for a confrontation. This is usually how people interpret this gesture. The challenge is that this is not always true because,

on some occasions, it can mean that the person is feeling cold and trying to find warmth in the heat that comes off that part of his arms. Another example is this; when a person sits with his feet pointing towards the direction of the door, it could mean that he feels bored and wants to be at another place.

4. **Tone of voice;** Much more than what you say, how you say it matters. The tone of voice is one form of non-verbal communication that you may not know how vital it is and the exact role it plays until you have made a wrong use of it. When you speak to people, they listen to the tone of your voice, and if it doesn't tally with the message you are trying to pass across, it can cause some kind of defensiveness in them. For example, a proper salutation has a tone of voice, and this tone of voice is not confrontational in nature. The nature of the message and the condition under which you are communicating will play a major role in making sure that the message is conveyed and accepted as it should be.

How Non-Verbal Communication Can Go Wrong

It is one thing to know the importance of non-verbal communication in your interactions with people, its another thing to make sure that you are not passing the wrong signals to people, and a different thing to make sure that the other person does not get the wrong impression of you and the message you are trying to pass across. It is usually within the second and third types of non-verbal communication mentioned above that these errors come into play.

When there is a disconnect between what your non-verbal communication portrays and what you are saying with your mouth, there is every tendency that the person on the other end can begin to doubt the authenticity of your communication. If this happens over time, they most likely will begin to believe that they cannot trust you. This is a recipe for disaster because when this distrust begins to make its way into a relationship, the result is that the relationship begins to suffer in all aspects.

Picking Up and Understanding Non-Verbal Signals

These are the steps you need to follow if you are going to pick up, analyze and profitably understand/make use of non-verbal signals.

1. Have a keen eye for details. Most of these non-verbal signals are given off unconsciously, so there is every tendency that even the person you are looking at does not know what he is looking out for; the non-verbal cues he is giving off. In order to be able to make the most out of trying to read non-verbal communication, train yourself to start seeing beneath the surface and what is presented.

2. Do not just look out for one signal; instead, look out for a group of signals that suggest the same thing. For example, saying that a person is warming up for a confrontation simply because he folded his arm across his chest alone may not be the appropriate interpretation. Rather, to validate that fact, look out for other signs that suggest that he is up to what you think he is. For

example, if he is showing other signs of restlessness like tapping his foot on the ground, then you may want to take those two signs more seriously. The goal here is to learn how not to isolate one sign and decide that it means one thing, after all.

3. While still interacting with people, understand that non-verbal communication may not always be as accurate as you think it is. There is always that little margin that can mean that it may be accurate or not. Have this in mind and ensure that you always address non-verbal communication from this point of view, and while you are at it, please learn to trust your guts.

Improving Non-Verbal Communication

While we have seen that non-verbal communication is a very handy tool in your day-to-day communication with people, it is not always a perfect index for measurement. This is because while trying to read and understand non-verbal communication, many cues can be overlooked and many things that were not there can be implied at the same time. As you try to improve your non-verbal communication skills, there are a few things you need to take note of;

- Learn to focus mostly on the now. Most of the cues you will be trying to read are subconscious and are subliminally acted by the people who are acting them. This implies that most of the time, they may not even know that they are giving off certain cues that can be expository. In order for you to be able to pick these up, you need to learn how to be in the moment. Many things will skip your notice if, in the face of a conversation, you let your mind wander off to another place.

- Consciously work on developing your emotional intelligence levels. Non-verbal communication is an aspect of emotional intelligence, and this is where you will learn how to make sure that your non-verbal communications tally with what you say with your mouth. When you have a higher emotional intelligence level, there is every chance that you will become more attuned to what the people around you are feeling per time. This way, you become a better communicator, show empathy for the other person and also get them to trust you almost immediately because of how accurate you are with your body language.

- You also need to know that improving non-verbal communication takes time. There is no magic wand that you can wave and become a professional in the art overnight. You need to learn how to achieve this and keep practicing with the information you have received. This is how you get better at it and also how you develop your emotional quotient.

How to Use Body Language to Influence People

Below are some of the subliminal cues you can send off to people, and how you can use these cues to influence them. Bear in mind, though, that what is written here is not a rule of thumb. Different people will react to different cues in different ways, and it is up to you to be able to understand the scenario and know your best line of action.

Smile at first

This is one way to get people to warm up to you almost instantly. When you begin with a smile (a conversation with a loved one, or a meeting with a stranger), you get the person to begin to see you as hospitable, friendly/approachable, and also as the kind of person to be trusted. The smile tells them to let down their guards for one bit, and this is what the person will most likely start doing. Here is a caveat, though; while you try to make use of this tool, make sure that the smile you are giving them is genuine and does not seem like a forced one or a leer. These will cause the person to shut down on you almost instantly.

Lean in

This works best when you are in the middle of a serious conversation with a person and you want him to know that he has your full attention. All you need to do here is to lean in towards the person or incline the upper part of your body toward him. This will give him the impression that he has your complete attention and this is one feeling that you want the people you converse with to have at all times. This is because once he comes to the agreement that he has your utmost attention, it means that there is nothing more important to you than what he is saying right now, and this is a great way to lure him into the place where he begins to speak more. The more he speaks, the more information you can get.

Control your feet

We discussed earlier that when your feet are pointed in the direction of the door or the exit, it can be suggestive of the fact that you have other better things to do and other better places to be in. Since this is not what you want to achieve, you need to make good use of your feet. Make sure they are pointed in the direction of the person you are conversing with. This sends the cue that you are paying close attention to what he is saying.

Exert dominance with your posture

This is very necessary if you are in a place where it seems as though there may be a little contention about who the boss is, and you are trying to nip that little tendency in the bud. One simple way to get this done is by making sure that your body posture reinforces the fact that you are the one in charge, confident but not too cocky, attentive, but not overbearing. To achieve this, you may want to stand with your feet planted firmly on the ground with the both of them apart and approximately at shoulders' distance. You may also want to stand akimbo and make sure that your head is held high.

These tips can help you influence people and get them to act in a certain way, just with your body language.

Key Points from Chapter Two

- Body language is a subset of non-verbal communication, and it is the kind of communication in which physical behaviors (as opposed to words) are used to express or convey information.

- Body language is almost as effective as verbal communication in interacting with people because most times, they give a clear insight into what you may be thinking or feeling at every point in time.

- While body language is a great way to know what someone thinks and feels, it may not be the ultimate test because it can be learned, and you can also learn to control your body language. The better you get at emotional intelligence, the easier it becomes for you to control and master your body movement.

A Short message from the Author:

Hey, I hope you are enjoying the book? I would love to hear your thoughts!

Many readers do not know how hard reviews are to come by and how much they help an author.

I would be incredibly grateful if you could take just 60 seconds to write a short review on the product page of my book from where your purchased a copy, even if it is a few sentences!

Thanks for the time taken to share your thoughts!

Chapter 3

Controlling People through Persuasion

What is Persuasion?

Persuasion is the process through which a person's attitudes, actions, and thought processes are influenced by another, especially without duress (Encyclopedia Britannica). Persuasion is dependent on communication and a lot more factors, including verbal threats, physical coercion, playing on one's psychological states and a whole lot of other elements.

Under these conditions, people are not exactly coerced; they are, however, influenced to see things through the lens of the person who is persuading them to go in a given direction. They reserve the right to execute what they are being persuaded to do or not.

Persuasion is only made possible as a result of influence. The person who is being persuaded into doing something must be under the influence of the one who is persuading – at least to some extent. This influence is usually what defines the hold the other has on him, and if this influence is not there, then there would not be any persuasion. For example, a boss that persuades his subordinate in the office to be an accomplice as he tells a lie to a board of directors banks on the knowledge of the fact that he wields a reasonable amount of influence on the subordinate whose life he can make better or worse depending on how well he is able to corporate with him to get him what he wants.

Persuasion, however, is not always used for all the bad reasons. As we have said time and again, it is completely dependent on the person that is wielding it and for what purpose he is wielding the influence.

Elements of Persuasion

Psychologists and experts on these matters generally agree that there are five elements of persuasion, and all of these play a strategic role in the process. Here is a quick rundown of them all.

1. The Source refers to the origin of the persuasion. This refers to the person or organization that is sponsoring the persuasion process, and for this

process to be successful, the source must be credible. There is an amount of trust and influence that must have been built by the source if they are going to be able to wield the powers of persuasion over anyone or any other organization. This influence and credibility are what make them worth being listened to in the first place.

2. The message is the information that the source wishes to pass over to a group of people and have them act on. This could be his ideologies, a concept he wishes them to adopt, or an action he wants them to carry out. If the message is not clear enough, then the source will not be able to drive action because the people on the other end will not know what he wants them to do.

3. The medium is as important as the message. This speaks of how the message is delivered to the people whom the source seeks to get a reaction out of. Understanding the medium is one of the criteria that will determine whether or not the

message will be delivered correctly and if the people on the other end will comply with what the source wants them to do. Some people argue that direct and spoken forms of communication are more effective in this process, but even in the absence of those, a lot more media can be used to influence and persuade people to move in a given direction. However, the goal of the message is that it must remain as concise as it can get so that the people who are supposed to be taking action on it can adapt immediately and make the needed changes they need to.

4. The audience speaks of those who are expected to receive the message from the source and move in a given direction. The success of this whole process depends on how they are able to assimilate the message and how willing they are to move in the direction the source wants them to move. This is why it is necessary for the source to understudy the audience for a while and understand what works for them and how he can

be able to get what he wants out of them. A lot is dependent on this factor.

5. The effect or the bottom line speaks of the action which the source wants his audience to take. This is the summary of the whole matter. The source must be able to take a look at the results he wants to gain and make sure that the audience is able to do what he intends for them to do. This feedback should be monitored at all times by the source if he is going to get the results he wants to get from the audience.

Manipulation Vs. Persuasion: The Thin Line

There is a very thin line that separates manipulation from persuasion, and if you don't know the boundaries, you may be tempted to swing into the other side of manipulation without your knowledge. This, sadly, has happened to many people and they ended up getting into what they were not supposed to get into without their own knowledge. The first thing you must learn in this section is that manipulation and persuasion are similar but are separated by a very thin line. Although they are similar, they can have polar opposite effects on people if used on them.

Here are a few short differences between the two.

1. **The intent;** According to a study carried out and documented in jonathanfields.com, this is unarguably the major difference between them. Manipulation is done with the sole intent to fool someone, control the person's actions completely and without letting him have a say in what he does, and also with the intentions of keeping the real implications of his actions away from him until the deed has been done. Manipulation is usually a dark process, and the end is that the person that is being manipulated will get into something he would not have otherwise done, especially without his knowledge of the full impact of his actions.

   Persuasion, on the other hand, is a bit less intense than this. Persuasion requires the will of the person involved because although you may be influencing his thoughts, he still has what it takes to say yes or no to what you are suggesting. Think of manipulation as covering the person's eyes with a blindfold and leading him through a hallway, while persuasion is more like taking the blindfold away and urging him to walk with you. In the first scenario, he has little or no idea of what he is really doing, but in the second scenario, he does.

2. **The benefits involved;** Manipulation is majorly carried out because the person carrying it out understands that there is so much he stands to gain if things are to go well, and the other person in the equation stands to gain very little as against the much he will gain, or may have nothing in it at all for him. Because people are generally hardwired to look out for their own personal interests, he understands that the other person may not be inclined to helping him get what he wants if he truly understands that there may be nothing in the deal for him. As a result of this, the person may be inclined to resort to devious means to get what he wants.

Persuasion, on the other hand, is usually mutually beneficial. For example, if you are looking to buy a product from a vendor but you are not sure which one to buy because there are a host of options available for you to choose from, the vendor can persuade you to get one. This is because, in either case, there are mutual benefits for both of you; he gets his money and you get a great product that will get you to come back sooner or later for another.

Subliminal Persuasion: How it Works

Have you ever been in a position where you needed someone to do something for you, and it was as though he was not inclined toward doing it at all, regardless? Perhaps you begged and pleaded with him to help you get that favor done, but all these were to no avail. If you have ever been in this situation and you finally got him to do that thing you wanted him to without the use of force (and without him telling you some spiritual forces urged him to help you, of course), then you probably made use of this technique. That's the interesting part; you may have used it even without your knowledge.

So, the real question now is, what is subliminal persuasion and how exactly does it work?

In a nutshell, subliminal persuasion is simply the art of persuading or influencing people to do something or move in a given direction by affecting them at a level that is lower than their normal conscious recognition (SocialMediaToday). It makes use of covert techniques and methods that cannot be easily spotted by the person on the receiving end.

Most of the techniques we have covered so far in this book are techniques that are not too hidden. Although they are not too glaring either (in the sense that one does not walk up to you and scream into your face that he is manipulating you), with a trained eye, you will be able to see when there is something wrong about the way someone relates with you. On the other hand, in this technique, special attention is paid to make sure that the modes of approach and the language/methods used in persuasion are undercover and not easily recognizable.

In today's world, almost everyone makes use of this method of persuasion at some point. The salesman trying to sell you his ware, or the preacher trying to convert you to his beliefs and religion all make use of this skill. Now that you know, let us take a quick look at how this works.

1. The first subliminal signal you send off to people is with your appearance. Your appearance has a lot to say to the people around you about your personality. Under these conditions, your appearance can be used as a tool to get you the attention you need and start eliciting the feelings you want to play upon as you interact with people. For example, if you are looking to appeal to the empathy or people's sense of pity, you may want to start out with looking the part. A lowly look will help you out with this. On the other hand, if you are looking to project confidence, attitude, and class, you must know what outfit to pull on. This is the first sign you send off to people and as the saying goes, first impression matter.

2. Start and lead the conversation. This sends over the signals that you are confident of what you are saying and that you are not afraid of navigating the conversation. This will come in very handy if you are looking to get a quick response out of the other person (especially if this response would have taken time to come, for example, to get him to make a buying decision immediately).

3. Lead with a clear and very firm voice. If you speak with a voice that wavers, it is indicative of insecurity or some form of fear and you do not want the other person to begin to read those signs. Be sure to apply this as a salesperson trying to get a prospect to patronize your business. In order to pull this off, you need to have a clear understanding of the product/service you are trying to sell and why the person on the other end of the exchange needs it. This knowledge will come in handy as it will be projected in your speech, mannerisms and in the confidence with which you communicate. Also, inflections and

your intonation will make all the difference in a conversation.

4. Subliminal persuasion requires that you are able to make quick and exact assumptions and sometimes conclusions about the person/people you are trying to win over. Make quick inferences about what they like and steer them in that direction. They will start feeling good about you and that is a very great subliminal persuasion tool. For example, you can get your prospective client a little gift. This way, he will be almost likely to hire you when he has the need for your products/services.

5. Subliminal persuasion makes use of presuppositions or assumptions. So, instead of asking open-ended questions, the person pulling this off makes use of questions that have been tailored to make sure that the person responding will give a certain kind of answer. For example, the person may ask "where would you want us to go on our NEXT date?" instead of "will you go

out with me again?" when he is trying to woo a lady. This way, she is almost unable to resist his advances towards her.

Subliminal persuasion is a great tool for convincing people to do something without getting them to feel too pressured. A good grasp of this will be great as you keep interacting with people.

Persuasion Techniques to Change Anyone's Mind

Here are a few of the techniques of persuasion that are used to change people's minds and how they work.

1. **Use of force (coercion);** This is probably the worst form of persuasion because it takes away the other person's sense of independence and the ability to choose. Coercion has been discussed in-depth in the preceding chapters.

2. **Creating a need (scarcity);** This tool is usually used by businesses and was also very common in medieval times. It is simply a situation in which a person or group of people at the helm of affairs as regards a situation, enforce compliance from the

masses by making sure that their supplies run out. For example, if a business is looking to increase the prices of one of their products, they can make use of this technique by stopping production. The sudden exit of the product from the marketplace will cause a demand that will reflect in the way the people will begin to look for the product. When the demand is at its height, they can reintroduce the product at a reviewed and higher price and because of the scarcity of that product in the past months, people will most likely have no option than to buy at the given rate. This is one of the most-used ways of ensuring that people comply with what others want; create a need that will force them to be interested in what you want them to be and introduce the product.

3. **Social proof;** This is another persuasion technique that is used mostly in business. It is anchored on the belief that people will be prone to believe something if there are witnesses to the fact that whatever is being said is true. Social

proof is any of such witnesses or statements made by a witness to corroborate the fact that something is true and that it works. For example, you are more likely to buy a product if you see testimonials as to its efficacy from other people. The testimonials lower your doubts and they are the social proof you need in order to make a buying decision.

4. **The foot in the door technique;** This principle is based upon testing the waters before taking a dive. It is all about starting small and gaining momentum as you go. In this technique, the user starts off the journey of persuasion by first asking for smaller favors, before the bigger ones. The idea is to butter the other person up for what he is about to ask for and have the person respond in a positive way. For example, "pass me the salt shaker," can be a foot in the door for "can you sign my recreation trip pass, please?" the child begins by asking the parent for smaller things, and the bigger things fall into place as time passes.

5. **The door in the face technique;** In a nutshell, this is the opposite of the technique discussed in the last point. Here, the person begins by asking you to do something that is too huge you know it is impossible and while you are still reeling from the impact of his request and refusing to get on with it, they ask you to help them achieve what they really wanted you to (which is a smaller task when contrasted against the other. The idea of this technique is to get you to do something by creating a picture in your mind as to how minute or little what they have requested for is when compared to what they asked you to do at first.

Resisting Persuasion Tactics Used By Manipulators

Once you have identified that you are being manipulated or forced to do something you would not have done otherwise, here is how you get yourself out of that position;

1. Have a clear understanding of what the word "NO" means, why you have said it and how to stand by your decisions once they are made. One

of the easiest things manipulators do is that they make you feel bad for saying NO to them. If you are able to pass through this step, you will stop feeling bad when you decline someone's request or decide that you cannot save everyone. Another thing to remember here is that you cannot save everyone, and even if you accept to do everything everyone asks for, it would still not be enough.

2. Know your fundamental human rights. This will help you to identify when someone is doing something that infringes on your rights, and you will be able to seek justice.

3. Deal with self-blame. When the manipulator does not get his way, it is only typical for him to want to play the blame game and try to make you feel bad for not permitting him to do what he wanted to do. He will try to play all cards that make you feel as though you have made a huge mistake, but remind yourself that you are not on a mission to walk through "blame street" many times a day.

4. Do not make major decisions when you are under duress, feel overwhelmed or when it looks as though there is more to an issue than meets the eye. Whenever you think you are being manipulated to do something, you may want to try turning the spotlight on the person you feel is manipulating you by beginning to ask them probing questions about what it is they want to do. If you find them slinking away and trying to act all shady, probably, what they wanted to do was not as innocent as they would have wanted you to believe it was.

Key Points from Chapter Three

- Persuasion is a skill that many people have wielded in order to get their ways with others. There are many forms of persuasion and it can be presented under a lot of facades, but the goal is still the same; to get someone to do what he was not going to do otherwise.

- There are 5 elements of persuasion and if the process is to be complete and yield the results the source wanted it to yield, all 5 elements must be in place.

- The gap between manipulation and persuasion is so thin that it is easy for you to find yourself slipping over to the place of manipulation (especially the wrong side of this) even without your knowledge. Know what separates both of them and set boundaries for yourself.

- As you walk through life on a daily basis, you are going to meet with people who will want to use manipulation to get you to do whatever they want you to do. A few tips have been discussed and these tips can help you break out from under their influence. Make use of these tips for your good.

Chapter 4

Neuro-linguistic Programming (NLP)

What is NLP

NLP is the process of analyzing and critically going through the strategies used by successful individuals and applying them to yourself in order to reach a personal goal (Goodtherapy.org). NLP is a psychological process and it involves critical analysis, observation of patterns and habits that are responsible for people's successes and also the adoption of the mindsets they have that has allowed them to achieve the goals they have achieved. When you are able to amass these information and tools, you apply them to your life and use them to further your ambitions or get yourself to the actualization of the goals you have set for yourself.

NLP seeks to find the relationship that exists between patterns of thoughts, languages and behavior to specific outcomes and results of enviable success.

The History Behind NLP

The history of NLP can be traced back to as far as the 1970s, and the relationship that existed between two scientists; Richard Bandler and John Grinder. Both of them worked in different faculties of the same institution and were astute scholars. They both had a vision and a burning desire to further their education and for personal development.

In pursuit of their success, they became curious because there was one thing that seemed to stand out for them; they wanted to know why certain people turned out successful against all the odds while the others seemed not to be able to achieve their dreams of success, regardless of what they tried. To be able to achieve this, they began to study in closer detail the lives of successful people that had lived before themselves. In carefully analyzing this, they began to discover a few parallels; there were some things that seemed to be constant with all these successful people regardless of what field they were succeeding in.

Drawn in by this discovery, they decided to adopt what they had seen so far and applied it to their lives. Just as the saying goes, *success leaves clues,* and in no time, these men began to experience drastic changes in their lives. More than just applying these to themselves, they began to incorporate them into their workshops and training as they taught a good number of students what they had learned so far. The students that went through the haggles of practicing what they were taught began to see the results in their lives as their successes began to increase on all fronts. This gave rise to a lot of interest in this area as notable scientists of the time began to take an interest in the subject matter.

Over the years, the subject of NLP has been undergoing a lot of expansion as a lot has been added to the mix, but it still subscribes to and goes to prove a point that sometimes, *you do not need to reinvent the wheel.* (Landsiedel NLP training)

How NLP works

Now that you know the history of NLP and what it is all about, it is time to take a brief look at how this works.

1. NLP is based on the belief that if a person can be able to understand how other successful people work and what is at the back of their successes, that he can be able to model that success and get the same result for himself.

2. NLP is unique to everyone. Those who propose the use of NLP believe that this is a unique pathway and that every human being has a specialized way in which they look at the world and the things that surround them. As a result of this, NLP is better suited to be applied by everyone individually, as there seems not to be a general approach to it.

3. Successful NLP begins with careful and close attention to details. Those who practice NLP start by analyzing themselves and the lives of the people who are successful and have gone way

ahead of them. The aim of this is to make sure that they are able to draw inferences and see where there are gaps that they must work on filling up immediately.

4. The NLP user gains information when he starts out on this journey of observation and close learning. This information begins to form the basis of all that he will begin to apply from the time he wants to see a change in aspects of his life.

5. When they have gained new information, the next step is that they must begin to apply all that they have learned. NLP instructors believe that the best way of learning is by practicing, and as a result of that, they are firm believers that after the learning comes the practice that will produce the results that they seek to have.

6. With the information the person has gathered, and the results of action, he can begin to seek therapy and the personal guide of his tutor. At this stage, the tutor begins to work with the

student under bespoke conditions and the result of this is that the student will usually begin to record massive growth in his life.

7. Drawing from the lessons he has learned from the successful people that are ahead of him, the student then begins to make alterations in his life where necessary. He starts working on his mindset, approach to life, habits and every other part of him that may be standing in the way of his success. In place of the limiting behaviors and mindsets he has been functioning with, he begins to adopt new ways and thought patterns. The result of this is that over time, he will begin to notice that there is marked and positive change/growth in his life.

How Effective is NLP

NLP is very effective, but this depends on a few factors.

1. How they are used

2. Who uses them. The student plays a major role in ensuring that NLP will work for him or

otherwise. He must be willing to put in the work required to get the results he wishes to see, or there would be nothing for him to celebrate.

3. Under what conditions they are used. NLP is not some form of magic. The student and the tutor alike must understand what makes NLP work and what conditions trigger their success or failure. Also, NLP is effective when the student is considered as a single entity and not as a community of students. This implies that NLP works more when they are used individually on students as this will help the coach to better understand what is needed by each student and how to channel his resources to make sure that the student succeeds.

NLP is generally effective and is applied in many places as discussed below.

Applications of NLP

1. In therapy. This is necessary to ensure that the therapist has a clear understanding of the person in therapy, has a working knowledge of his unique challenges and can address all the issues that made him report to the clinic. Since all that can be used are foundational knowledge in various sectors (as different things may make sense to different people), it is necessary that the therapist understands NLP. This way, he can establish a connection with his patient and be able to come up with a special plan to make sure that the patient becomes better. Over time, NLP have been used to handle cases like Schizophrenia, PTSD, stress, and many other related issues.

2. NLP can be applied in sociological interactions of people and is a very great background knowledge that can help you become apt at reading body language. For example, with your knowledge of NLP, you are able to detect cues that people give off faster than the person that

does not have a working knowledge of NLP. This way, you can be better prepared for challenges that may arise in social settings.

3. NLP can be used in career advancements. When you understudy the lives of those that have gone ahead of you, you can be able to learn something you would not have otherwise known. This way, you begin to position yourself for career advancement and the opportunity to become better.

Techniques Used in NLP

Here are a few NLP techniques that can help you get started on the path of achieving what you want to achieve with your life (thelawofattraction.com)

Reframing

Just as the name implies, reframing is the art of changing your perspective and deciding to see things from a different lens, from a positive lens rather than from a negative standpoint. Reframing is a healthy way to make sure that you do not get struck down when challenges come to you, but that you are able to chart a course out of problems that may flood your path. Simply put, reframing is taking the negative things that happen to you, looking at them from a positive light, and with the energy that comes from there, making your way forward.

For instance, if you fail a course and have to repeat a class in a school, rather than having to look at it as some big misfortune, you can see it as an opportunity to get to know what you did not know before in a better way, and also perform your best the next time. This way, you feel inspired and ready to take charge of your success.

Self-anchoring

This is the process by which you get the desired positive emotional responses with a particular occurrence, phrase or feeling. Choosing a positive emotion or feeling and associating it with a little gesture that you perform every now and then will ensure that you always feel good because, as you carry out this gesture, you get to release all the good feelings that you have come to associate with it. For example, you can anchor the feeling of being productive and in control of your day with something as little as brushing your teeth or making your bed in the morning. This way, whenever you are carrying out this act, you can begin to feel these empowering feelings as they begin to well up within you.

Dissociation

This is a simple technique of separating yourself emotionally and psychologically from experiences that leave a bitter taste in your mouth. Things tend to hurt you all the more because you are in the present and you feel the pain of whatever happens to you as it begins to happen. Dissociation, however, allows you the luxury of pulling yourself out of bad situations and observing like a spectator. The next time you are faced with an ugly circumstance and you are at the edge of giving up, close your eyes and imagine yourself floating out of your body to watch what is happening as a spectator. After a few short minutes of being in this position, you will begin to notice changes in your attitude and this will help you begin to see things from a clearer perspective and make adjustments where necessary.

Building rapport

This is simply the use of a predetermined set of body language to send over a message to another person's psyche that you care for him and that you are a likable person. In the preceding sections, we have talked about these body languages that can get people to like you faster. You may want to pull them out and begin to practice them.

How to Use NLP to Persuade Others

Here are a few tips to help you make use of NLP to persuade people to do what you want them to do. These tips are going to draw from what has been discussed in other sections of the book and seeing as we have thrown light in those sections, this section will be brief.

1. Dress like an influencer. Remember that one of the non-verbal cues people pick up about you is tied up in how you dress. If you are looking to get

people to listen to you, you must look like someone that is worth being listened to.

2. Listen to people more than you talk. This allows you to be able to pay attention to even what is not being said and draw inferences from there. Also, this tip helps people believe that you are genuinely interested in them and they will begin to open up to you all the more.

3. Employ the correct use of body posture as you interact with people. This will make sure that they feel comfortable with you, and this is the first step to using NLP to get what you want.

4. Be open with people. They do not need to feel that you are trying to hide something away from them. If they do, they will start feeling closed-off and you don't want this happening to you if you want to win them over.

Protecting Yourself from NLP Mind Control

1. Take a closer look at people who copy your body language. They most likely are up to something and being aware of that can help you reinforce your mental shields.

2. Minimize body contact with people. As we said earlier, one of the ways people project themselves on you is with bodily contact. In order to reduce this risk, make sure that people do not get to touch you a lot – especially people you do not know and trust.

3. Pay attention to language. Those who make use of NLP to control others are very good at making use of vague, ambiguous and permissive language. The goal is to get you to fall into a trap, after which they can bait you into doing something you would not have done. In order to reduce the likelihood of this happening to you, close off all communication when you begin to notice this and take your exit. You may want to continue later or not, but do not be there.

4. With those you think are trying to pull this stunt (NLP mind control) on you, make sure you are always at attention when you are around them. Spacing out on them is literally you handing them an olive branch to jump in on your psychology and do what they want to do with it within the minutes you space out. It may not be as easy as you think, but it will save you a lot of stress as time proceeds.

5. In times like these, you have to learn to trust your gut feeling. This may not have any logical explanation and may not be able to be explained away by science, but it is one thing that will help save you a lot of stress. If your gut feeling says no to a thing, try to leave it at that or at least give more time to think it over. You would be saving yourself a lot of trauma.

Key Points from Chapter Four

- NLP is the study of patterns, habits and mindsets of successful people with the sole intent of applying these to your life in order to reach a goal and become more successful.

- NLP has many applications, including in therapy, business and personal development.

- You will meet people who will try to make use of NLP to influence you to do things you may not want to do. You need to make it a point of duty to spot these ones out and erect defenses to make sure that they never get their way with you.

The end... almost!

Hey! We've made it to the final chapter of this book, and I hope you've enjoyed it so far.

If you have not done so yet, I would be incredibly thankful if you could take just a minute to leave a quick review on my book product page.

I would be incredibly grateful if you could take just 60 seconds to write a short review on the product page of my book from where your purchased a copy, even if it is a few sentences!

Even if it is just a sentence or two!

So if you really enjoyed this book, please...

Leave a brief review on on the product page of my book from where your purchased a copy.

I truly appreciate your effort to leave your review, as it truly makes a huge difference.

I truly appreciate your effort to leave your review, as it truly makes a huge difference.

Chapter 5

Influencing Others with Mind Control

What is Mind Control?

Mind control, also known as brainwashing, is the process by which individual or collective freedom of choice and action is compromised by agents or agencies that modify or distort perception, motivation, cognition or behavioral outcomes (Wikipedia). Simply put, brainwashing is the process by which a person's ability to think for himself and make informed decisions is taken away from him by another person and, most times, not exactly through the use of force.

Mind control is usually accomplished over a long period of time. As opposed to other forms of influencing people, which are usually almost instantaneous and yield results that can be seen in the short run, brainwashing usually takes a longer amount of time to be achieved and when it has taken its full course, it can produce very lethal results. Mind control can also be referred to as coercive persuasion, thought control or thought reform.

How Does Mind Control Work?

1. Mind control starts from the place where the perpetrator of this act breaks the person he is trying to brainwash down. He does not do this by beating him with a stick; rather, he achieves this aim by getting the person to a place where he is mentally at his weakest.

   During the course of history, many cult groups have risen up and some of them have thrived for a very long time. This is one thing that almost all of these groups have in common, and it is the absolute power and influence of the leader over the people that are following him. The leader is usually able to achieve this aim by brainwashing the people and getting them to a point where they get to see him as the absolute authority figure over their lives. In this scenario, breaking down a person will usually take these forms;

- The person gets exposed to something he has never been exposed to all his life. It could be love, or affluence, or shows of affection and attention; the goal is to get this person to begin to feel as though there is a lot that he has missed out on all his life.

- After a very short season of enjoying these benefits, the person will have to return to his normal life. Because of the fact that what he has tasted is much better than what he has in his life, a repulsion for that life will begin to rise within him.

- Suddenly, there will be a reappearance of the person who is trying to brainwash the other. He may resurface at any time and this time, he will make sure to make the person he wants to get into his net feel special, properly attended to and the center of his world. This unlocks a lot of feelings that will get the other person to be trapped and insanely attracted to the rush of good emotions that come with being that person at the center of another's world.

- At the nick of time, he will begin to buttress on points that are sore for the person he is trying to brainwash. He can begin to throw light on what is wrong in the person's life and how he feels because of all the things he has been made to pass through. Normally, this will open up a lot of emotions and this is the point where the person looking to brainwash slips in with his devious craft.

2. The next step is usually to introduce a 'solution.' At the point the person who is being brainwashed begins to feel emotionally drawn and broken, the person who is performing the act on him swoops in like the knight in shiny armor he is projecting himself to be and provide unsolicited answers.

   It could be an emotional boost to make him feel better, or the promise of a good life afterward, but the rationale is to make the person an offer that sounds too good to be true.

3. Brainwashing thrives on the presence of peer pressure. Once the leader has introduced his solutions, it is very likely that the person he is trying to get onboard will not accept them immediately. This is all good because all it will take will be a short while until the person has to make a definitive choice, whether to get on board or to disembark fully. Since it is highly probable that almost all the people in that sect have the same mindset, the person who is being brought onboard will have no choice than to begin to give special thought to the proposition he has received.

4. Brainwashing at this level is highly successful because of a few reasons;

- Social isolation; the leader most likely has created a community where he assembles his followers and they interact together as a closely-knit community.
- Information control; this is probably the most important factor in the equation. There has to be

a system of making sure that what the people hear is consistent with what the leader wants them to hear. The leader takes it upon himself to feed them with what he wants them to hear, and this is done consistently and over a long period.

5. After this, there is a system of reinforcement that is put in place. This is the guarantee that people will continue to believe what the leader is saying and his ideologies.

This system of brainwashing has been used over the years, especially by cult groups. It is the reason why the followers believe in things that seem to be too ridiculous and can stake their lives on them. A quick example of such cult group was The order of the Solar temple founded in the late 1790s – early 1980s by Frenchmen Luc Jouret and Joseph Di Mambro.

When is Mind Control Useful?

Mind control can be useful under the following situations;

1. In technology and as new technological devices geared towards making life easier begin to hit the market.

2. When you want to make a request of someone and the person is most likely not going to accept what you are requesting for.

3. Some elements of mind control can be handy when you are looking to pull people together to achieve a common aim.

Generally, scientists and other people believe that mind control may be an extreme form of influencing people's psychology and should be avoided as much as possible.

Techniques Used in Mind Control

Here are a few mind control techniques that have been used to brainwash people in the past. The aim of this list is to get you to be aware of these techniques and know when people around you are trying to use them on you.

Isolation

This is usually the bedrock of mind control. All mind control and brainwashing exercises are largely dependent on how successful the isolation process goes. This is one thing that was common for all the cult groups that were mentioned in the section above; there was a system for isolating people. Physical isolation is a very functional mind control technique and even when it is not possible for physical control, the person who is trying to brainwash another does all he can to isolate him emotionally, mentally and in every wise. The aim of this step is to cut him off from the real world so that he can have his way with him.

Peer pressure and social proof

These are other techniques that have been used to brainwash people. Social proof is the psychological phenomenon in which people assume that the actions and beliefs of others are appropriate and since 'others do that,' the action is justifiable (psychologia.co). Peer pressure can also be a viable technique because the person's free will is most likely to be taken when he sees that all his peers are up to the same thing and has no choice other than to join them.

Repetition
Whatever you are going to be brainwashed into believing and ultimately acting upon has to be repeated to you over and over again before it sinks well enough into your mind and you believe it as much as the person who is brainwashing you wants you to.

The new identity concept and the severing of natural ties
When someone is about to brainwash you, he makes up a new identity for you (and this is not in the healthy, empowering way that you know). The new identity is usually something completely foreign from what you knew and believed about yourself. The aim of this is to create an identity that is manipulated by them, and if they are able to achieve this, they will move on to make sure that they severe all your natural ties. Brainwashers usually achieve their aim by pulling those that are brainwashing away from their natural habitat, influence them to let go of their family and friendship ties. This

way, they become entirely new beings and in the wrong way.

Criticism

This is employed as the manipulator t=or the person who initiates the brainwashing begins to criticize and make everything that is not initiated by himself look as though they are wrong and will be detrimental to the person he wants to influence by brainwashing.

Signs You are Being Brainwashed

Here are a few red flags that may suggest that you are being brainwashed

1. You most likely are being brainwashed if you rely heavily on the validation and approval of the person who is brainwashing you. In the business world, the equivalent of this is if your annual performance review in your workplace is a very big event in your life and you cannot wait for it. (Forbes.com)

2. You are most likely being brainwashed if you never question the decisions and actions of the

person who is brainwashing you, even when it is evident that what he is doing is wrong.

3. When you begin to desire the attention and affection of any sect or people who you are not supposed to be desirous of these attention and affection from. This is a clear sign that you are getting emotionally attached and being brainwashed inadvertently.

4. You are most likely being brainwashed if, in an exchange or interaction with a person, he keeps repeating something as though it were a mantra and he is expecting you to believe it as he says it is. This may be a great time to seek a way to put a stop to that conversation or you may end up falling for what he is saying.

5. You are likely being brainwashed at work if you feel guilty for needing tools and facilities to aid your work and help you with your productivity.

Defending Yourself from Mind Control Manipulation

In the last chapter, we discussed how you can be able to defend yourself from NLP mind control, and those points apply even in this context. In addition to those points that were discussed,

1. Develop your cognitive abilities. One of the ways to avoid being brainwashed is to develop an independent mind. With this mind, you can be able to find out what is wrong and not be afraid to question things you feel are not right.

2. Have a clear vision. Chances of being swayed from side to side will greatly reduce when you have a clear vision for your life, career, relationship and even your intentions. This closes any loophole for the person who wants to brainwash you to slip in from.

3. Take time to establish healthy relationships with the people around you and in your life. Reach out to your friends and family and make sure you have someone you can confide in should in case things begin to spiral out of control.

4. Set boundaries for yourself and make sure to remain within the confines of the boundaries you have set for yourself. While you are at it, know when to push forward and when to take a step back from the situations you find yourself in.

5. Look out for subliminal cues as they have been discussed in this book and nip them in the bud once you see them.

Getting What You Want Using Mind Control

Here are a few ideas that can help you when you are looking to obtain something from someone, and you are in need of getting them to answer in the affirmative.

1. Do your best to take away their thinking power from them. Although this may sound devious, one of the biggest mistakes you can make is to ask who you want to obtain something from to think it over. The chances are that if he is to do just that, he will begin to see cracks in what you want him to do and this will make him develop cold feet. So, if you are selling a product, do your

best to help your prospect make an immediate buying decision.

2. When you are about to make a request, start with something small but make sure that you go beyond what you asked for. For example, if you want to sell a car to a worker who probably has to live off of a budget, do not start by pitching yourself to him as the owner of a car dealership; he will most likely run away from you at first sight. You can start by offering him good advice on how to manage the car he is presently using or even sell to him the break fluid his mechanic needs to fix the car. From there, you can then start pitching the new car to him, starting with why he needs a new car and how cost-friendly it will be in the long run for him to save the money he has been spending on fixing the old car. With this, you start implanting yourself in his mind and he will be sure to come to you when he is going to get a new car.

3. Give a lot more than you take. This is a law of life; you cannot be a parasite and expect that people will love you and feel comfortable around you. To get close enough to people, be that one person who gives to make the lives of others better. With this, you get people to be open to you and it is a great start for you to have access to them.

4. Do not be afraid to ask for what you want straight-up. This act sometimes will throw the person off-balance and you may find him giving in to your request just because you caught him off-guard. Another reason for this is because sometimes, you need to come off as straight-to-the-point and not-beating-about-the-bush to be able to get the respect and attention of the person.

5. Add to this list what you have learned from NLP and you will be well on your way to making the most out of every opportunity and getting people to answer favorably to all your requests or most of them.

Key Points from Chapter Five

- Mind control is the process by which individual or collective freedom of choice and action is compromised by agents or agencies that modify or distort perception, motivation, cognition or behavioral outcomes.

- Mind control can be a tool of mass destruction and has been in existence and active use over the years.

- There are many mind control techniques, including isolation and social proof. You must train yourself to see through these and get yourself away from those that try to make use of mind control against you. At the same time, there are a few techniques that you can apply that will help you as a person; in your business, personal life and career. Find these in the preceding sections and be sure to include them when next you are going to make a request.

Conclusion

You meet with different people every day, and not all these people have your best interest at heart.

Some of them are devious people who would not hesitate to walk all over you in order to get what they want for themselves.

Others may be good but subconsciously making use of tricks and skills that are like a double-edged sword to get what they want from you, not knowing that they may also be misusing these skills while at it.

You may even be the one making use of these techniques to get what you want. In any case, this book has been written to serve as a guide for you.

In the preceding pages, you have learned different concepts and how they all coagulate towards advancing your social life or pulling it back. In the last few pages you have learned how to speed read people from the cues they give off with their bodies, how to influence the people around you and also protect yourself from the harmful influence of those that try pulling a few bad stunts on you.

Be sure to go over what you have learned in this book. Commit to heart all the key notes touched on and from your interaction with the knowledge contained in this book, draw action points you can get started on immediately. It is all about how you are able to put in practice all you have learned.

Cheers to a better and wiser you!

References

Lee, J., 2014. The Human Dark Side; Evolutionary Psychology and the Original Sin. Retrieved from; https://link.springer.com/article/10.1007/s10943-013-9805-z

Islahi, A. A., March 1993. Good and Evil (2): View of the Qur'an. Retrieved from http://www.al-mawrid.org/index.php/articles/view/good-and-evil-2-view-of-the-quran

Murphy, B., December 2015. 11 psychological tricks to manipulate people, ranked in order of pure evilness. Retrieved from; https://www.inc.com/bill-murphy-jr/evil-psychological-tricks-to-manipulate-people.html

Wikipedia.com., N.d. The Dark Triad. Retrieved from https://en.m.wikipedia.org/wiki/Dark_triad

Barrios, J., N.d. 10 ways manipulators use emotional intelligence for evil (and how to fight back). Retrieved from https://www.inc.com/justin-bariso/10-ways-manipulators-use-emotional-intelligence-for-evil-and-how-to-fight-back.html

Wikia.org., N.d. Body Language. Retrieved from
https://psychology.wikia.org/wiki/Body_language

Silverman, J., September 2000. Remember the five basic
elements of persuasion. Retrieved from
https://www.bizjournals.com/albany/stories/2000/09/25/
smallb5.html

Hurst, K., N.d. what is NLP? 5 techniques that will
transform your life. retrieved from
https://www.thelawofattraction.com/5-nlp-techniques-
will-transform-life/

Ryan, L., May 2016. Ten unmistakable signs you are
brainwashed. Retrieved from
https://www.forbes.com/sites/lizryan/2016/05/15/ten-
unmistakable-signs-youre-brainwashed/amp/

Printed in the USA
CPSIA information can be obtained
at www.ICGtesting.com
LVHW010242201123
764398LV00004B/377